RESISTANCE BANDS WORKOUTS FOR SENIORS:

Effective Resistance Band Workouts at Home or on the Go to improve Strength and Balance

BY

JORGE FRIEL

TABLE OF CONTENTS

INTRODUCTION

Aging is an inevitable part of life, a natural journey we all embark upon. As we grow older, we find ourselves facing new challenges, experiencing changes in our bodies, and confronting various health concerns. For seniors, maintaining an active and healthy lifestyle becomes increasingly vital, not only for prolonging their years but also for enhancing their overall quality of life. In this pursuit, resistance bands emerge as a remarkable and invaluable tool that can help seniors combat the effects of aging and improve their physical well-bcing.

Resistance bands, sometimes referred to as exercise bands or resistance tubing, are elastic bands made from various materials such as rubber, latex, or fabric. They come in a range of resistances, allowing individuals to tailor their workouts to their specific needs and abilities. While resistance bands have gained popularity in recent years among fitness enthusiasts of all ages, they hold particular promise for seniors seeking to maintain their strength, flexibility, and mobility.

The aging process is often associated with a decline in muscle mass, a decrease in bone density, and an increased risk of chronic health conditions like osteoarthritis and diabetes. These challenges can lead to a reduced ability to perform daily activities, a loss of independence, and an overall diminished quality of life. However, the good news is that regular exercise, including resistance band training, can be a powerful antidote to many of these age-related issues.

In this exploration of resistance bands for seniors, we will delve into the numerous physical and psychological benefits that these versatile tools offer. From strengthening muscles and improving balance to enhancing cardiovascular health and promoting mental well-being, resistance bands have the potential to revolutionize the way seniors approach fitness and aging. Furthermore, we will provide a comprehensive guide on how to get started with resistance band exercises, ensuring that seniors can incorporate this beneficial practice into their daily routines with ease and confidence.

Join us on this journey of discovery as we uncover the multifaceted advantages of resistance bands for seniors. Through a combination of scientific research, expert insights, and real-life success stories, we will illustrate how these unassuming elastic bands can empower older adults to lead healthier, more active, and fulfilling lives. So, let's embark on this enlightening journey to better understand the incredible benefits that resistance bands bring to the lives of seniors, opening doors to a world of improved physical well-being, increased confidence, and enhanced longevity.

CHAPTER 1: GETTING STARTED WITH RESISTANCE BANDS

Selecting the Right Resistance Bands for Your Needs

Resistance bands have become increasingly popular for their versatility, affordability, and effectiveness in providing a full-body workout. Whether you're a beginner looking to kickstart your fitness journey or an experienced athlete wanting to add variety to your routine, resistance bands can be a valuable tool. However, selecting the right resistance bands is crucial to achieving your fitness goals safely and effectively. This guide will help you get started on the right foot.

Understanding Resistance Bands

Resistance bands are flexible, stretchy bands that come in various shapes, sizes, and levels of resistance. They work by adding resistance to your exercises, allowing you to target specific muscle groups or perform full-body workouts. These bands are suitable for various fitness goals, including strength training, muscle toning, rehabilitation, and enhancing flexibility.

Before diving into the selection process, it's essential to understand the different types of resistance bands:

Loop Bands: These are continuous, closed-loop bands that come in various resistance levels. They're excellent for lower body exercises, such as squats and lunges.

Tube Bands with Handles: These bands consist of a tube with handles on each end. They are versatile and can be used for a wide range of upper and lower body exercises.

Flat Bands: These are thin, flat strips of latex or fabric. They are primarily used for lower body exercises and stretching routines.

Figure-8 Bands: These bands are shaped like the number eight and are designed for specific exercises targeting the arms, chest, and shoulders.

Choosing the Right Resistance Level

Selecting the appropriate resistance level is crucial to ensure that your workouts are challenging but achievable. Resistance bands typically come in various color-coded levels:

Light (Yellow or Green): Ideal for beginners, rehabilitation, and those looking to enhance flexibility.

Medium (Red or Blue): Suitable for intermediate users or those seeking a balance of strength and flexibility.

Heavy (Black or Purple): Designed for advanced users or those looking to build muscle and strength.

It's essential to start with a resistance level that matches your current fitness level. As you progress, you can gradually move up to higher resistance bands to keep challenging yourself.

Factors to Consider

When selecting resistance bands, consider the following factors:

Material: Latex is the most common material used for resistance bands, but there are latex-free options available for those with allergies. Ensure that the material is durable and won't snap easily.

Quality: Invest in high-quality bands that won't wear out quickly. Look for brands that offer a warranty to ensure their durability.

Handles and Accessories: If you're choosing tube bands with handles, make sure the handles are comfortable and secure. Some bands come with door anchors and ankle straps for added versatility.

Length and Size: Ensure the bands are the right length for your intended exercises. Longer bands provide more versatility but may be less convenient for certain exercises.

Portability: Consider whether you need bands that are easy to transport for workouts on the go.

Safety: Always inspect your bands for any tears, cracks, or signs of wear before using them. Use them on a stable surface to prevent accidents.

Getting Started

Once you've selected the right resistance bands, you can begin incorporating them into your fitness routine. Start with basic exercises and gradually increase the intensity and complexity as you become more comfortable. Online tutorials and fitness apps can provide guidance and workout routines tailored to your goals.

Resistance bands are an excellent addition to your fitness arsenal, offering a wide range of exercises and benefits. By choosing the right bands and using them safely, you can embark on a rewarding fitness journey that aligns with your goals and preferences. Remember to consult a fitness professional or physical therapist if you have any specific health concerns or limitations.

Safety Precautions and Proper Technique

Resistance bands are versatile and effective tools for strength training and rehabilitation. They provide resistance in various directions, allowing you to target different muscle groups and adapt to your fitness level. Whether you're a beginner or an experienced fitness enthusiast, incorporating resistance bands into your workouts can offer a host of benefits. However, it's essential to use them safely and with proper technique to avoid injury and maximize your results. In this guide, we'll explore safety precautions and the correct techniques for getting started with resistance bands.

Safety Precautions:

Inspect Your Bands: Before each workout, examine your resistance bands for any signs of wear and tear. Check for cracks, fraying, or any visible damage. If you find any issues, it's crucial to replace the band to prevent injury.

Proper Anchor Point: When using resistance bands, ensure they are anchored securely. A sturdy door anchor or attachment point designed for resistance bands is recommended. Avoid using objects that may shift or break under tension.

Choose the Right Resistance Level: Resistance bands come in various levels of resistance. Start with a light resistance band if you're new to strength training and gradually work your way up to heavier bands as you become stronger.

Warm-Up: Always perform a thorough warm-up before using resistance bands to prepare your muscles and joints for the workout. This can help reduce the risk of injury.

Maintain Proper Form: Good form is essential for both safety and effectiveness. Keep your movements controlled and precise to target the intended muscles and prevent strain on joints. Engage your core muscles to stabilize your body.

Control the Band: As you perform exercises, maintain control over the band's tension. Letting the band snap back uncontrollably can lead to injuries. Slow and controlled movements are key.

Avoid Overstretching: Resistance bands can be stretched up to a certain point, but avoid overstretching them beyond their limit, as this can cause them to snap back and potentially harm you.

Proper Technique:

Start Slowly: If you're new to resistance bands, begin with simple exercises like bicep curls, squats, or shoulder presses to get used to the equipment.

Use Full Range of Motion: Utilize the band's resistance throughout the entire range of motion in each exercise. This ensures you engage the muscles effectively and avoid unnecessary strain.

Breathing: Remember to breathe properly during your exercises. Exhale during the effort phase and inhale during the relaxation phase of the exercisc. This helps with both performance and safety.

Variety of Exercises: Resistance bands can be used for a wide range of exercises, including chest presses, rows, leg lifts, and more. Incorporate variety into your routine to target different muscle groups and prevent overuse injuries.

Consult a Professional: If you're unsure about the right techniques for your specific goals or have any concerns about using resistance bands, consider seeking guidance from a fitness professional or physical therapist.

Progressive Overload: To continually challenge your muscles and make progress, increase the resistance level of your bands as your strength improves. This gradual progression is essential for long-term gains.

Incorporating resistance bands into your fitness routine can be a game-changer. They are cost-effective, portable, and adaptable, making them an excellent choice for home workouts or when you're on the go. By following these safety precautions and mastering proper techniques, you'll minimize the risk of injury and maximize the benefits of resistance band training, helping you reach your fitness goals more effectively.

Setting Realistic Goals and Tracking Progress

Resistance bands are versatile and effective tools for building strength, toning muscles, and improving flexibility. Whether you're a beginner or an experienced fitness enthusiast, setting realistic goals and tracking your progress is essential to stay motivated and see tangible results. In this guide, we'll explore how to get started with resistance bands, establish achievable fitness goals, and monitor your advancements along the way.

Getting Started with Resistance Bands

Before diving into goal-setting and tracking progress, it's important to familiarize yourself with resistance bands and their benefits:

Types of Resistance Bands

There are various types of resistance bands, including loop bands, tube bands with handles, and figure-eight bands. Each type offers different levels of resistance and versatility for various exercises. Choose the one that suits your needs and preferences.

Benefits of Resistance Bands

Portable: Resistance bands are lightweight and easy to transport, making them an excellent choice for home workouts, travel, or taking to the gym.

Versatile: You can use resistance bands to target almost every muscle group in your body, making them suitable for both strength training and flexibility exercises.

Low Impact: They are gentle on the joints, reducing the risk of injury compared to heavyweights.

Suitable for All Levels: Whether you're a beginner or an advanced athlete, resistance bands can be adjusted to provide the right level of challenge.

Now that you're equipped with the basics, let's move on to setting realistic fitness goals.

Setting Realistic Goals

Define Your Objectives: Start by understanding what you want to achieve with resistance bands. Are you looking to build muscle, increase your endurance, or improve your flexibility? Having a clear objective will guide your training program.

S.M.A.R.T. Goals: Make your goals Specific, Measurable, Achievable, Relevant, and Time-bound (S.M.A.R.T.). For example, "I want to lose 10 pounds in 3 months by incorporating resistance band workouts into my routine."

Know Your Current Level: Assess your current fitness level. Knowing where you are will help you set realistic goals. It's okay to start with beginner exercises and gradually progress.

Consult a Professional: If you're new to resistance bands or have specific fitness goals, consider consulting a fitness trainer or physical therapist. They can provide guidance tailored to your needs.

Create a Plan: Develop a workout plan that includes a variety of exercises targeting different muscle groups. A well-rounded routine will help you achieve your goals more effectively.

Monitor Progress: Keep a workout journal to track your workouts, including the type of exercises, resistance levels, and repetitions. This will help you stay on track and make necessary adjustments.

Tracking Progress

Tracking your progress is essential to stay motivated and make informed decisions about your resistance band workouts:

Record Measurements: Take initial measurements of your body, such as weight, body fat percentage, and circumferences of key areas. Periodically reassess these measurements to see changes over time.

Track Repetitions and Resistance Levels:
Maintain a detailed log of the exercises you perform, the number of repetitions, and the resistance levels used. As you get stronger, increase the resistance gradually.

Assess Your Strength: Periodically test your strength by trying to lift heavier resistance bands or perform more repetitions. This will help you gauge your progress and set new goals.

Evaluate How You Feel: Pay attention to how your body feels and any improvements in your overall fitness, such as increased energy levels, reduced pain, or enhanced flexibility.

Celebrate Milestones: When you reach specific milestones or achieve your S.M.A.R.T. goals, celebrate your accomplishments. Reward yourself to maintain motivation.

Adjust Your Plan: Based on your progress, make necessary adjustments to your workout plan. If a particular exercise becomes too easy, increase the resistance or try more challenging variations.

In conclusion, getting started with resistance bands is an excellent way to improve your fitness and strength. Setting realistic goals and tracking your progress will keep you motivated and ensure that you are on the path to success. Remember that consistency and dedication are key to achieving your fitness aspirations with resistance bands.

CHAPTER 2: STRENGTH-BUILDING WORKOUTS

Upper Body Strength and Endurance Exercises

A strong and resilient upper body is not only essential for athletic performance but also for everyday activities and overall health. Upper body strength and endurance workouts are crucial for improving posture, preventing injuries, and enhancing your ability to perform daily tasks with ease. In this guide, we'll explore a variety of exercises that will help you build upper body strength and endurance. Whether you're an athlete aiming to enhance your performance or someone looking to improve their overall fitness, this comprehensive workout routine is for you.

Push-Ups:

Push-ups are a classic upper body exercise that engages your chest, shoulders, triceps, and core. They can be modified to suit your fitness level. Start with standard push-ups and progress to decline or incline push-ups for added intensity.

How to do it: Begin in a plank position with your hands slightly wider than shoulder-width apart. Lower your body until your chest nearly touches the ground, then push back up to the starting position.

Pull-Ups:

Pull-ups are an excellent exercise for strengthening your back and biceps, enhancing your grip strength, and increasing upper body endurance. If you're new to pull-ups, consider using an assisted pull-up machine or resistance bands to make them more manageable.

How to do it: Hang from a pull-up bar with your palms facing away from you. Pull your body up until your chin is above the bar, then lower yourself down with control.

Dips:

Dips target the triceps, chest, and shoulders. You can do these using parallel bars or a sturdy surface like the edge of a bench or the back of two stable chairs.

How to do it: Place your hands on the bars or surface with your arms fully extended. Lower your body by bending your elbows, then push back up until your arms are straight.

Bench Press:

Bench presses are a fundamental exercise for building chest and tricep strength. You can do this exercise with a barbell or dumbbells.

How to do it: Lie on a bench, hold the barbell or dumbbells above your chest, and lower them to your chest before pushing them back up.

Plank:

While planks are often seen as a core exercise, they also engage the shoulders, chest, and upper back. Planks are fantastic for building endurance and stability.

How to do it: Start in a push-up position but with your weight supported on your forearms. Keep your body in a straight line from head to heels, engaging your core muscles throughout.

Rows:

Rowing exercises, whether with resistance bands, dumbbells, or a cable machine, are ideal for developing upper back strength, enhancing posture, and preventing imbalances.

How to do it: Hold the handles or weights in front of you, and pull them towards your lower ribcage while squeezing your shoulder blades together.

Incorporating these upper body strength and endurance exercises into your workout routine can help you achieve a well-balanced, robust upper body. Consistency and gradual progression are key to seeing improvements in strength and endurance. Remember to warm up before starting your workout and to cool down and stretch afterward. It's also essential to maintain proper form and, if necessary, seek guidance from a fitness professional to ensure you're performing these exercises correctly and safely. Building upper body strength and endurance is not only about aesthetics but also about overall health and functional fitness, so make it a priority in your fitness journey.

Lower Body Strength and Stability Exercises

A strong and stable lower body is the foundation for overall strength, balance, and functionality. Whether you're an athlete aiming to enhance your performance, a fitness enthusiast looking to build muscle, or simply someone who wants to improve their daily life, lower body strength and stability exercises are essential. In this guide, we'll explore a variety of effective exercises that target your lower body, helping you achieve greater strength and stability.

Benefits of Lower Body Strength and Stability Exercises:

Improved Muscle Strength: These exercises engage major muscle groups in the lower body, such as the quadriceps, hamstrings, glutes, and calves, resulting in increased muscle strength and definition.

Enhanced Balance and Coordination: Incorporating stability exercises helps improve balance and coordination, reducing the risk of falls and injuries.

Greater Athletic Performance: Athletes can benefit from lower body workouts to enhance their speed, agility, and power, crucial for various sports and activities.

Enhanced Daily Functionality: A strong lower body makes daily activities like walking, climbing stairs, and carrying groceries more manageable and less physically demanding.

Lower Body Strength and Stability Exercises:

Squats:

Stand with your feet shoulder-width apart.

Lower your body by bending your knees and pushing your hips back.

Keep your back straight and your chest up.

Push through your heels to return to the starting position.

This exercise targets the quads, hamstrings, and glutes.

Lunges:

Step forward with one foot and lower your body until both knees are bent at a 90-degree angle.

Ensure your front knee does not extend beyond your toes.

Push back to the starting position.

Lunges work the quads, hamstrings, and glutes while improving balance.

Deadlifts:

Stand with your feet hip-width apart and a barbell in front of you.

Bend at your hips and knees to lower your torso while keeping your back straight.

Grip the barbell and lift it while keeping it close to your body.

Return to the starting position.

Deadlifts primarily target the hamstrings, glutes, and lower back.

Leg Raises:

Lie on your back with your arms by your sides.

Lift one leg off the ground and keep it straight.

Hold for a few seconds and lower it back down.

Repeat with the other leg.

Leg raises help strengthen the hip flexors and lower abdominal muscles.

Bosu Ball Squats:

Stand on a Bosu ball with the flat side down.

Perform squats as you would on solid ground.

The unstable surface engages the stabilizing muscles in your lower body.

Step-Ups:

Use a sturdy platform or bench.

Step onto the platform with one foot and push through the heel to stand up.

Step back down and repeat on the other leg.

Step-ups strengthen the quads, hamstrings, and glutes while improving balance.

Incorporating lower body strength and stability exercises into your fitness routine is essential for a well-rounded and robust physique. These exercises not only help you build muscle but also improve balance and coordination, which are vital for daily life and athletic performance. Whether you're a fitness enthusiast or an athlete, the exercises listed above can be tailored to your specific needs and goals, providing a solid foundation for lower body strength and stability.

Core Strengthening for Improved Posture and Balance

A strong and stable core is the foundation of a healthy body. It not only gives you the sculpted abs many desire but also plays a crucial role in maintaining good posture and balance. Core strengthening workouts are not just about aesthetics; they are about overall health and well-being. In this article, we'll explore the importance of core strength, the benefits it offers, and how to incorporate core-focused exercises into your fitness routine to enhance your posture and balance.

The Importance of Core Strength

Your core encompasses the muscles in your abdomen, lower back, and pelvis. These muscles work together to provide stability for your spine, hips, and pelvis. A strong core is essential for various daily activities, including standing, sitting, lifting, and even maintaining balance during simple tasks.

Benefits of Core Strengthening

Improved Posture: A strong core provides the support needed to maintain an upright posture. When your core muscles are weak, it's common to slouch or hunch over, which can lead to poor posture. By strengthening your core, you can help alleviate or prevent posture-related issues, such as lower back pain and rounded shoulders.

Better Balance: A stable core is vital for balance and coordination. Strong core muscles enable you to react more effectively to changes in your body's position, reducing the risk of falls and injuries, especially as you age.

Enhanced Athletic Performance: Whether you're a seasoned athlete or a fitness enthusiast, a strong core is essential for performance in various sports and activities. It allows for more efficient power transfer and movement, helping you excel in your chosen field.

Lower Back Pain Relief: Core strength is often prescribed as a solution for lower back pain. Strengthening the core can provide relief by providing better support to the spine and reducing the strain on the lower back.

Core Strengthening Exercises

Incorporating core strengthening workouts into your routine is essential for reaping the benefits of improved posture and balance. Here are some effective exercises to get you started:

Planks: The plank is a classic core exercise that engages the entire core, from your abs to your lower back. Start in a push-up position, resting on your forearms and toes, and hold the position as long as you can.

Russian Twists: Sit on the floor with your knees bent and your feet flat. Lean back slightly and lift your feet off the ground. Hold your hands together and twist your torso to each side, touching the ground next to your hip.

Leg Raises: Lie on your back with your hands under your hips. Lift your legs, keeping them straight, until they are perpendicular to the floor, then lower them back down without touching the ground.

Bridges: Lie on your back with your knees bent and your feet flat on the floor. Lift your hips off the ground, forming a straight line from your shoulders to your knees.

Superman Pose: Lie face down with your arms and legs extended. Lift your arms, chest, and legs off the ground simultaneously, engaging your lower back and glutes.

Core strengthening workouts are a vital component of any fitness routine, offering a myriad of benefits beyond aesthetics. A strong core is key to maintaining good posture, improving balance, preventing injuries, and enhancing overall well-being. By incorporating core-focused exercises into your workout regimen, you can enjoy a healthier, more balanced life while standing tall with confidence.

Remember to consult with a fitness professional or healthcare provider before beginning any new exercise program, especially if you have pre-existing medical conditions or concerns.

CHAPTER 3: BALANCE AND FLEXIBILITY EXERCISES

Enhancing Balance and Stability for Fall Prevention

Maintaining balance and flexibility is crucial for individuals of all ages, but it becomes increasingly vital as we get older. Falls are a significant concern for seniors and can lead to serious injuries and a loss of independence. To combat this issue, incorporating balance and flexibility exercises into your routine can make a substantial difference in enhancing your overall stability and reducing the risk of falls. In this article, we will explore the importance of these exercises in fall prevention and provide some practical tips for incorporating them into your daily life.

The Importance of Balance and Flexibility

Fall Prevention: According to the World Health Organization, falls are the second leading cause of accidental injury and death worldwide, with adults aged 65 and older being particularly susceptible. Maintaining good balance and flexibility can significantly reduce the likelihood of falling.

Improved Quality of Life: Balance and flexibility exercises help improve overall mobility, making it easier to perform everyday tasks and maintain an active, independent lifestyle. Enhanced balance and stability also boost self-confidence.

Injury Prevention: Good balance and flexibility can help prevent injuries not only from falls but also from everyday accidents. When you can move with ease and maintain equilibrium, you are less likely to strain or sprain muscles or joints.

Balance Exercises

Balance exercises are designed to improve your ability to control your body's position, either in static or dynamic situations. Here are some simple exercises to enhance your balance:

Single Leg Stands: Stand on one leg for 30 seconds or longer. Repeat on the other leg. You can hold onto a sturdy chair for support if needed.

Heel-to-Toe Walk: Take small steps, placing the heel of one foot directly in front of the toes of the other. Walk in a straight line for about 20 steps.

Tai Chi: Consider joining a Tai Chi class. This ancient Chinese martial art focuses on slow, flowing movements that promote balance, flexibility, and strength.

Flexibility Exercises

Flexibility exercises help improve the range of motion in your joints and reduce muscle stiffness. Here are some flexibility exercises to consider:

Stretching: Incorporate daily stretching routines for major muscle groups. Focus on your neck, shoulders, back, hips, thighs, calves, and ankles.

Yoga: Regular yoga practice is an excellent way to improve flexibility, balance, and overall well-being. Many yoga classes are designed with seniors in mind, emphasizing gentle, accessible postures.

Pilates: Pilates focuses on core strength and flexibility, making it an effective choice for those seeking improved stability.

Incorporating Balance and Flexibility Exercises into Your Routine

Start Slow: If you're new to balance and flexibility exercises, begin with easy, low-impact activities and gradually increase the intensity and duration as your abilities improve.

Consistency is Key: Aim to incorporate these exercises into your daily routine. Consistency will yield the best results.

Professional Guidance: Consult with a healthcare professional or physical therapist to create a personalized exercise plan that suits your needs and considers any pre-existing health conditions.

Social Support: Consider engaging in these exercises with friends or joining a class specifically designed for seniors. Social support can motivate you to stay active.

Balance and flexibility exercises are integral to maintaining overall health and well-being, especially for seniors who wish to prevent falls and injuries. By incorporating these exercises into your daily routine, you can significantly enhance your stability, mobility, and quality of life. The investment in your physical health will pay off, allowing you to continue living an active, independent life with confidence.

Increasing Flexibility and Range of Motion

Achieving balance and flexibility is not only essential for athletes and dancers but is also crucial for individuals of all ages and fitness levels. It plays a vital role in maintaining overall health and well-being. As we age, our flexibility tends to decrease, making everyday activities more challenging. However, with the right exercises and a consistent routine, you can increase your flexibility and range of motion, improving your quality of life. This article will delve into the importance of balance and flexibility exercises and provide you with a range of effective exercises to help you achieve your flexibility goals.

The Importance of Balance and Flexibility

Injury Prevention: Enhanced flexibility reduces the risk of injuries, especially during physical activities and sports. It enables your joints and muscles to move more freely and adapt to unexpected movements.

Posture Improvement: Better flexibility can help maintain good posture, reducing the risk of developing musculoskeletal problems. It also relieves tension in your muscles and joints.

Enhanced Range of Motion: Improved flexibility allows you to move your joints through a wider range of motion, making everyday activities easier and more comfortable.

Stress Reduction: Balance and flexibility exercises can promote relaxation by reducing muscle tension and promoting the release of endorphins.

Better Performance: Athletes and individuals who engage in sports can enhance their performance by increasing their flexibility, allowing for more agility and efficient movements.

Balance and Flexibility Exercises

Yoga: Yoga is a versatile and popular practice that combines balance, strength, and flexibility exercises. It involves various poses, stretches, and breathing techniques to promote flexibility and balance.

Pilates: Pilates focuses on core strength and flexibility. It's an excellent way to improve your balance and flexibility through controlled movements that target specific muscle groups.

Stretching: Incorporate regular stretching routines into your daily schedule. Dynamic stretches before exercise and static stretches afterward can improve flexibility over time.

Tai Chi: Tai Chi is a slow and graceful form of exercise that enhances balance, flexibility, and mental focus. It's particularly beneficial for older adults.

Resistance Training: Resistance exercises using bands or weights can strengthen the muscles and improve joint stability, indirectly contributing to better flexibility.

Balance Exercises: Simple balance exercises like standing on one foot, heel-to-toe walks, and balancing on a stability ball can significantly improve your overall balance and stability.

Foam Rolling: Myofascial release through foam rolling can help reduce muscle knots and improve flexibility. Roll slowly over tight muscles to release tension.

Active Isolated Stretching: Active isolated stretching involves holding a stretch for a short duration, releasing, and then repeating. It can help increase flexibility without the risk of overstretching.

Tips for a Successful Flexibility Routine

Warm up before stretching to prepare your muscles for greater flexibility.

Breathe deeply and focus on relaxing into each stretch.

Progress gradually and do not force your body into extreme positions.

Consistency is key; regular practice will yield better results over time.

Listen to your body. If you experience pain during a stretch, back off to avoid injury.

Balanced and flexible muscles and joints are essential for overall health and vitality. Incorporating balance and flexibility exercises into your daily routine can enhance your quality of life by reducing the risk of injuries, improving posture, reducing stress, and enhancing your performance in physical activities. Remember to start slowly, be patient with your progress, and make flexibility training a regular part of your fitness routine to reap the many benefits it offers.

Stretching Routines to Relieve Tension and Aches

Maintaining a healthy lifestyle isn't just about cardiovascular workouts and strength training; it also includes balance and flexibility exercises. These often overlooked components of fitness are crucial for overall well-being, injury prevention, and relief from tension and aches. In this article, we will explore the importance of balance and flexibility exercises and provide you with some effective stretching routines to incorporate into your fitness regimen.

The Significance of Balance and Flexibility

Injury Prevention: Balance and flexibility exercises are essential for injury prevention. They help improve your range of motion, reduce muscle imbalances, and enhance your body's ability to adapt to various physical challenges, reducing the risk of sprains, strains, and falls.

Pain Relief: Many people suffer from chronic aches and pains, often stemming from tight muscles and poor posture. Regular stretching and balance exercises can alleviate these discomforts by increasing blood flow, reducing muscle tension, and promoting relaxation.

Improved Posture: Poor posture is a common problem in today's sedentary world. Balance and flexibility exercises can help correct imbalances, promote an upright posture, and reduce the strain on your spine and supporting muscles.

Enhanced Athletic Performance: Whether you're an athlete or just an active individual, improved flexibility and balance can enhance your performance. Better flexibility leads to a greater range of motion, while better balance helps with stability and agility.

Effective Stretching Routines

Static Stretching: This involves holding a stretch in a fixed position for 15-30 seconds. Perform static stretches for major muscle groups such as the hamstrings, quadriceps, calves, and shoulders. Ensure you maintain proper form and avoid bouncing, which can lead to injury.

Dynamic Stretching: Dynamic stretching involves moving your muscles and joints through their full range of motion. Activities like leg swings, arm circles, and hip rotations are excellent examples. Dynamic stretching is ideal for warming up before exercise.

Yoga: Yoga is a comprehensive system that combines flexibility, balance, and strength. Many yoga poses focus on enhancing flexibility and balance, making it an excellent addition to your routine. Sun Salutations, Downward Dog, and Warrior Poses are great choices.

Pilates: Pilates emphasizes core strength, posture, and flexibility. Incorporating Pilates exercises into your routine can help improve balance and flexibility while toning your muscles.

Tai Chi: Tai Chi is a gentle martial art that focuses on balance and flow. Its slow, deliberate movements are perfect for enhancing balance and reducing tension. Consider joining a Tai Chi class or following instructional videos.

Foam Rolling: While not a traditional stretching routine, foam rolling helps release tension in muscles through self-massage. Foam rollers are particularly effective for loosening tight areas like the IT band, quadriceps, and lower back.

Tips for a Successful Stretching Routine

Warm up before stretching to prepare your muscles and joints for the exercises.

Breathe deeply and consistently during stretches to relax your muscles.

Be patient and gradual in your approach. Don't force your body into uncomfortable positions.

Incorporate balance exercises like single-leg stands or tree poses to improve stability.

Stretch regularly, ideally incorporating these exercises into your daily routine.

Balance and flexibility exercises are vital for achieving a well-rounded, healthy lifestyle. They promote injury prevention, pain relief, better posture, and enhanced athletic performance. By incorporating stretching routines and balance exercises into your fitness regimen, you can reap these benefits while achieving a greater sense of well-being and vitality. So, whether you're a fitness enthusiast or a beginner, start making balance and flexibility a part of your daily life for a happier and healthier you.

CHAPTER 4: FULL-BODY WORKOUTS FOR SENIORS

Combining Strength, Balance, and Flexibility

Staying active and maintaining a healthy lifestyle is essential at every age, and for seniors, it's especially important. Full-body workouts that focus on strength, balance, and flexibility can help older adults lead a more independent and fulfilling life. These workouts not only improve physical well-being but also enhance mental and emotional health. In this article, we'll explore the benefits of full-body workouts for seniors and provide a sample exercise routine to help you get started.

The Importance of Full-Body Workouts for Seniors

Strength: Maintaining muscle strength is vital for seniors, as it aids in daily activities such as carrying groceries, getting up from a chair, and preventing falls. Strength training can improve bone density and help combat age-related muscle loss, making seniors more resilient.

Balance: Balance exercises are crucial to prevent falls, which can lead to serious injuries. A strong core and leg muscles are essential for stability and can help seniors maintain their independence.

Flexibility: As we age, our joints tend to stiffen, reducing our range of motion. Flexibility exercises can counteract this effect, helping seniors remain agile and reducing the risk of injury.

Sample Full-Body Workout Routine for Seniors

Always consult with a healthcare professional before starting a new exercise regimen, especially if you have underlying health concerns. Start slowly and progress at your own pace, focusing on proper form and safety.

Warm-Up (5-10 minutes):

March in place or walk around your home to increase blood flow.

Arm circles and leg swings to loosen up your joints.

Gentle neck stretches and deep breaths to relax.

Strength Training (2-3 times per week):

Bodyweight squats: Stand with your feet shoulder-width apart and squat down as if you're sitting in a chair. Do 2 sets of 10-12 reps.

Wall push-ups: Place your hands on a wall, shoulder-width apart, and push yourself away from the wall. Do 2 sets of 10-12 reps.

Leg lifts: Hold onto a sturdy surface for support and lift one leg straight out to the side. Do 2 sets of 10-12 reps for each leg.

Balance Exercises (2-3 times per week):

One-legged stand: Stand on one leg and try to maintain your balance for 30 seconds to 1 minute. Switch to the other leg.

Heel-to-toe walk: Walk in a straight line, placing one foot in front of the other, with your heel touching your toe as you progress.

Flexibility Training (daily):
Neck and shoulder stretches.
Arm and wrist stretches.
Gentle spinal twists.
Leg stretches, including calf, hamstring, and quadriceps stretches.

Cool-Down (5-10 minutes):
Slowly walk around or march in place.
Stretching exercises targeting major muscle groups.
Deep breathing to relax and lower your heart rate.

Full-body workouts that combine strength, balance, and flexibility exercises are a great way for seniors to stay active and maintain their overall well-being. These workouts help improve muscle strength, balance, and flexibility, which are crucial for daily activities and fall prevention. Remember to consult with a healthcare professional before starting any exercise routine and always prioritize safety and proper form. Staying active can lead to a healthier, more independent, and fulfilling life for seniors.

Tailoring Workouts to Your Fitness Level

Maintaining an active lifestyle is crucial for seniors, as it can help improve overall health, increase mobility, and enhance the quality of life. Full-body workouts designed specifically for seniors can be a fantastic way to achieve these benefits. However, it's important to tailor these workouts to your fitness level to ensure safety and effectiveness. In this article, we'll explore the importance of full-body workouts for seniors and provide valuable tips on how to customize your routine to match your fitness level.

The Importance of Full-Body Workouts for Seniors

Full-body workouts for seniors offer a range of benefits that can enhance physical, mental, and emotional well-being. Here are some of the key advantages:

Enhanced Muscle Strength: As we age, we naturally lose muscle mass. Full-body workouts help seniors maintain and even increase muscle strength, making everyday activities easier.

Improved Balance and Coordination: Balance and coordination are essential for preventing falls and maintaining independence. Full-body exercises can help seniors develop better balance and coordination.

Increased Flexibility: Regular full-body workouts can improve joint flexibility, reducing the risk of injury and enhancing mobility.

Heart Health: Exercise is beneficial for cardiovascular health, helping to reduce the risk of heart disease, high blood pressure, and stroke.

Mental Well-being: Physical activity is known to boost mood, reduce stress, and improve cognitive function, promoting a positive outlook on life.

Tailoring Workouts to Your Fitness Level

The key to successful full-body workouts for seniors is to customize your routine to match your individual fitness level. Here's how to get started:

Consult with a Healthcare Professional: Before beginning any exercise program, it's essential to consult with your healthcare provider. They can assess your current health status and provide guidance on what types of exercises are safe for you.

Set Realistic Goals: Start with achievable fitness goals that are specific to your needs. Whether you aim to improve balance, build strength, or increase endurance, setting clear objectives will help keep you motivatcd.

Choose the Right Exercises: Based on your health assessment and goals, select exercises that suit your fitness level. These can include gentle forms of cardio, such as walking or water aerobics, and resistance exercises using light weights or resistance bands.

Prioritize Safety: Safety should be a top concern. Ensure that you have proper footwear, use assistive devices if needed, and exercise on a non-slip surface to prevent accidents.

Progress Gradually: As your strength and endurance improve, gradually increase the intensity and duration of your workouts. This progression will help you continue to see positive results without risking injury.

Include a Variety of Movements: Incorporate a variety of exercises that target different muscle groups and movements. This will provide a well-rounded full-body workout and prevent overuse injuries.

Listen to Your Body: Pay attention to how your body responds to exercise. If you experience pain, discomfort, or fatigue beyond what's normal, stop the activity and consult with your healthcare provider.

Full-body workouts for seniors offer a multitude of physical and mental benefits. By tailoring your exercise routine to your fitness level, you can enjoy these advantages while minimizing the risk of injury. Remember that the key to successful workouts is consistency and gradual progression. Seek guidance from healthcare professionals, set achievable goals, and embrace the positive impact that regular physical activity can have on your senior years.

Sample Workout Plans for Home and Travel

Staying active and maintaining a healthy lifestyle is crucial for seniors, as it can help improve strength, balance, and overall well-being. Full-body workouts for seniors are a great way to achieve these goals while enjoying the benefits of exercise. In this article, we'll provide sample workout plans designed for seniors that can be done at home or while traveling, ensuring that physical fitness remains a priority no matter the location.

Why Full-Body Workouts for Seniors?

Full-body workouts are essential for seniors because they target multiple muscle groups, promote flexibility, and help with balance. They also contribute to the prevention of age-related muscle and bone loss, ultimately enhancing independence and overall quality of life. These workouts can be adapted to individual fitness levels and needs, making them accessible to a wide range of seniors.

Sample Workout Plans

Home-Based Full-Body Workout for Seniors
This workout can be done in the comfort of your own home, requiring minimal equipment. It focuses on strength, balance, and flexibility.

Warm-Up (5-10 minutes):
- *March in place*
- *Arm circles*
- *Ankle circles*
- *Neck stretches*

Strength and Balance Exercises (20-30 minutes):

- *Bodyweight squats (10-15 reps)*
- *Wall push-ups (10-15 reps)*
- *Leg raises (10-15 reps per leg)*
- *Chair dips (10-15 reps)*
- *Planks (10-20 seconds)*

Cool-Down (5-10 minutes):

- *Gentle stretching for major muscle groups*
- *Travel-Friendly Full-Body Workout for Seniors*
- *If you're on the go or traveling, you can still maintain your fitness routine with minimal equipment. This workout focuses on bodyweight exercises that can be done in a small space, such as a hotel room.*

Warm-Up (5-10 minutes):

- *March in place*
- *Arm circles*
- *Ankle circles*
- *Neck stretches*

Strength and Balance Exercises (20-30 minutes):

- *Standing leg lifts (10-15 reps per leg)*
- *Wall angels (10-15 reps)*
- *Seated leg extensions (10-15 reps)*
- *Planks (10-20 seconds)*
- *Standing calf raises (10-15 reps)*

Cool-Down (5-10 minutes):

Gentle stretching for major muscle groups

General Tips for Full-Body Workouts for Seniors

Start Slow: If you're new to exercise or haven't worked out in a while, start with lighter weights or resistance and gradually increase as you get stronger.

Listen to Your Body: Pay attention to how your body feels during and after exercise. If you experience pain or discomfort, adjust or modify the exercises accordingly.

Stay Hydrated: Drink plenty of water before, during, and after your workouts, especially when traveling to different climates.

Consistency is Key: Try to stick to a regular workout schedule, even when on the road.

Consistency will help you maintain and improve your fitness level.

Consult a Professional: If you have any medical conditions or concerns, consult with a healthcare professional or a certified fitness trainer before starting a new exercise routine.

Full-body workouts for seniors are a wonderful way to maintain physical health and well-being, whether at home or while traveling. These sample workout plans can serve as a foundation for your exercise routine, and you can adjust them based on your individual needs and preferences. Remember that consistency and dedication are the keys to reaping the numerous benefits of regular exercise, helping you stay active, independent, and healthy as you age.

CHAPTER 5: STAYING CONSISTENT AND ADAPTING OVER TIME

Motivation and Staying Committed to Your Routine

Consistency is the key to achieving success in almost every aspect of life. Whether you're working towards your fitness goals, pursuing a career, or nurturing personal relationships, staying committed to a routine is vital. However, the path to success is rarely linear, and challenges and unexpected circumstances often require us to adapt. In this article, we will explore the importance of staying consistent and adapting over time to maintain motivation and commitment to your routine.

The Power of Consistency

Consistency is the foundation of progress. When you engage in a routine consistently, you build habits and momentum. These habits not only make it easier to accomplish tasks but also increase your confidence and self-discipline. Over time, they become an integral part of your life, reducing the mental effort required to maintain them.

Setting Clear Goals: Start by defining your goals. Whether it's achieving a fitness milestone, advancing in your career, or enhancing a skill, having clear, measurable objectives provides a sense of purpose and direction. Write down your goals and regularly revisit them to stay motivated.

Establishing a Routine: A routine provides structure and discipline. Create a daily or weekly schedule that incorporates the actions needed to work toward your goals. Stick to your routine as closely as possible, as consistency breeds success.

Accountability: Share your goals and progress with a friend or mentor who can help hold you accountable. Having someone to report to can boost your motivation and commitment.

Adapting to Challenges

Life is unpredictable, and obstacles are bound to arise. Adapting to these challenges without losing motivation is crucial.

Flexibility: Be open to adjustments in your routine when necessary. If an unexpected event disrupts your plans, adapt your schedule without guilt. Flexibility is not the enemy of consistency; it is its ally.

Learning from Failure: Instead of being disheartened by setbacks, use them as opportunities for growth. Analyze what went wrong, adjust your approach, and keep moving forward.

Patience: Understand that progress often occurs in waves. You may not see immediate results, but stay committed to your routine, and eventually, your efforts will pay off.

Self-Compassion: Be kind to yourself. It's okay to have off days or to make mistakes. Acknowledge your imperfections, but do not let them deter you from your goals.

Motivation Strategies

Staying motivated throughout your journey is challenging, but there are strategies to keep your enthusiasm alive.

Visualization: Imagine your success vividly. Visualizing the end result can serve as a powerful motivator, reminding you of the benefits of your consistent efforts.

Celebrate Milestones: Recognize and celebrate your achievements, no matter how small they may seem. Rewarding yourself for reaching milestones can boost motivation.

Surround Yourself with Positivity: Engage with positive and supportive individuals who inspire you to stay committed to your routine. Their encouragement can be a tremendous source of motivation.

Keep Learning: Continuous self-improvement and learning can reignite your passion for your routine. Stay curious and explore new aspects of your chosen path.

Staying consistent and adapting over time is a dynamic process that requires motivation and commitment. By setting clear goals, establishing a routine, and staying accountable, you can build a solid foundation for success. When facing challenges, flexibility, patience, and self-compassion will help you stay on track. Remember, the journey toward your goals is a marathon, not a sprint. Stay motivated, keep adapting, and success will be within reach.

Modifying Workouts as Your Fitness Improves

Consistency in your fitness routine is a vital component of achieving your health and fitness goals. However, as your fitness improves, it's equally important to adapt and modify your workouts to continue making progress and avoid plateaus. This delicate balance of staying consistent while also evolving your exercise regimen is key to long-term success in your fitness journey.

The Importance of Consistency

Consistency is the foundation of any successful fitness journey. It means committing to regular workouts and making exercise a part of your daily or weekly routine. Consistency helps you build healthy habits, increase your strength, and improve your overall fitness level over time. But staying consistent doesn't mean doing the same workout forever.

Adaptation as a Sign of Progress

As you become fitter and stronger, your body adapts to the exercise routines you've been following. This adaptation is a sign of progress, but it can also lead to diminished results if you don't change things up. To continue making gains in your fitness, you must be willing to adapt and modify your workouts. Here's how you can do that:

Progressive Overload: This concept involves gradually increasing the demands on your body to stimulate further adaptation. You can achieve this by adding more weight, increasing the number of repetitions or sets, or altering your exercise intensity.

Varied Exercises: Incorporate new exercises into your routine. For example, if you've been doing traditional bench presses for chest strength, consider adding incline bench presses or push-ups to target your muscles from different angles.

Change the Routine: Don't follow the same workout plan indefinitely. Create new routines every few weeks to keep your workouts fresh and challenging. This can prevent boredom and stimulate further progress.

Modify Rest Intervals: Adjusting the time you rest between sets can change the intensity of your workouts. Shorter rest periods can make your workouts more demanding, while longer rest periods can help you recover during particularly intense routines.

Nutrition and Recovery: As your fitness improves, your nutritional needs may change. Ensure that your diet supports your fitness goals and provides the necessary nutrients for recovery and growth.

Listen to Your Body: Pay attention to how your body responds to your workouts. If you consistently experience pain, fatigue, or decreased performance in a certain area, it may be a sign that it's time to adapt your approach.

The Benefits of Adaptation

Adapting your workouts as your fitness improves offers several benefits:

Preventing Plateaus: Regularly changing your exercise routines helps you avoid fitness plateaus, where your progress stagnates.

Reducing the Risk of Injury: By incorporating variety and listening to your body, you can reduce the risk of overuse injuries associated with repeating the same exercises.

Improved Motivation: Changing up your workouts can keep you motivated and excited about your fitness journey.

Balanced Development: Adapting your workouts can help you achieve a more balanced and well-rounded physique by targeting different muscle groups and movements.

Staying consistent with your fitness routine is crucial for making progress, but it's equally important to adapt and modify your workouts as your fitness improves. Embrace change and continue challenging yourself to reach new levels of strength and endurance. By doing so, you can ensure that your fitness journey remains rewarding, exciting, and free from plateaus. Remember, it's not about doing the same thing over and over; it's about evolving and growing with your fitness.

Incorporating Resistance Bands into Daily Life

In today's fast-paced world, maintaining a consistent fitness routine can be a real challenge. Between work commitments, family responsibilities, and various other daily tasks, finding time for the gym or regular workouts can be difficult. However, there's a versatile and convenient solution to help you stay consistent with your fitness goals: resistance bands. Not only do these simple yet effective tools allow you to stay on track, but they also offer room for adaptation and growth over time.

Why Resistance Bands?

Resistance bands have gained immense popularity in recent years for good reason. They are lightweight, affordable, and incredibly versatile, making them the ideal choice for people with busy schedules or those looking to diversify their fitness routine. Here's why resistance bands are an excellent addition to your daily life:

Portability: Resistance bands are compact and easy to carry, making it possible to exercise at home, in the office, or even while traveling. Their portability eliminates the need for expensive gym memberships or bulky exercise equipment.

Adaptability: Resistance bands come in various levels of resistance, from light to heavy. This means you can tailor your workouts to your fitness level and adapt as you become stronger over time. They also allow you to replicate various exercises performed with traditional gym equipment.

Low Impact: If you have joint issues or are recovering from an injury, resistance bands offer a low-impact option for strength training. They reduce the risk of strain and injury, making them suitable for people of all ages and fitness levels.

Comprehensive Workouts: Resistance bands can be used to target every muscle group, providing a comprehensive full-body workout. Whether you want to build muscle, improve flexibility, or increase endurance, resistance bands can help you achieve your fitness goals.

Incorporating Resistance Bands into Your Daily Life

Now that you know the benefits of resistance bands, it's time to explore how to incorporate them into your daily routine effectively.

Morning Stretch: Start your day with a gentle stretching routine using resistance bands. These bands can help you increase flexibility and mobility, preventing muscle stiffness and promoting good posture.

Quick Workouts: When time is limited, resistance bands are your best friend. You can squeeze in a short, effective workout during your lunch break or whenever you have a spare moment.

Home-Based Workouts: Design a small workout space in your home with a few resistance bands and incorporate them into your daily exercise regimen. You can do squats, lunges, bicep curls, and more right in your living room.

Outdoor Exercise: Take your resistance bands to the park, beach, or any outdoor location. Combine the beauty of nature with an efficient workout.

Progressive Training: As you become more comfortable with your resistance bands, gradually increase the resistance level to ensure continued growth and challenge in your workouts.

Family Fitness: Get your family involved! Resistance bands can be used by people of all ages, so consider family workouts to encourage a healthy, active lifestyle.

Staying consistent with your fitness routine and adapting it over time is crucial for achieving your health and wellness goals. Resistance bands are a practical and versatile solution to help you maintain your fitness journey, regardless of your schedule or experience level. By incorporating resistance bands into your daily life, you can enjoy the convenience, flexibility, and effectiveness they offer, ensuring that you stay on track and adapt to your evolving fitness needs over time. Make them a part of your daily routine, and you'll soon discover the positive impact they have on your health and well-being.

CONCLUSION

In conclusion, "Resistance Bands Workouts For Seniors" serves as a comprehensive guide to empower older adults on their journey towards improved strength and balance. Throughout the chapters, we have explored the versatility and effectiveness of resistance band workouts, offering a practical solution for seniors looking to maintain and enhance their physical well-being. As we reach the final pages of this book, it is essential to reflect on the key takeaways and the broader message it conveys.

First and foremost, the power of resistance bands lies in their accessibility. These simple yet versatile tools have provided seniors with a means of enhancing their fitness from the comfort of their homes or while on the go. They require minimal space and equipment, making them a cost-effective and convenient choice for individuals of all fitness levels.

Moreover, this book has emphasized the importance of tailor-made exercise routincs that cater to the specific needs and capabilities of seniors. The provided workouts, meticulously designed to target strength and balance, take into account the challenges and concerns that often accompany aging. By following these routines, seniors can expect not only physical improvements but also a boost in their confidence, overall well-being, and independence.

The chapters of this book have also highlighted the significance of consistency and dedication in the pursuit of health and fitness goals. Progress may not always be immediate, but with time and commitment, the rewards will manifest themselves in enhanced muscle strength, improved balance, and ultimately, a better quality of life. Each resistance band workout is a step toward a healthier, more active, and independent future.

Furthermore, the testimonials and success stories featured in this book have shown the real-life impact of resistance band workouts on the lives of seniors. The stories of resilience and determination serve as a testament to the transformative power of these exercises, proving that it is never too late to invest in one's health and well-being.

In closing, "Resistance Bands Workouts For Seniors" is more than just a fitness guide; it is a roadmap to a more vibrant and fulfilling life. By embracing the principles and exercises outlined in this book, seniors can embark on a journey to better health, greater strength, and enhanced balance. Remember that the path to improved well-being is within your reach, and with the right tools and dedication, you can make significant strides towards a healthier and more active future. It is our hope that this book has provided you with the knowledge, inspiration, and motivation needed to embark on this transformative journey. So, take your resistance bands, take that first step, and take charge of your health and happiness. Your journey begins now.